R. A. FORSTER F.I.M.L.S.
REGIONAL MYCOLOGY LABORATORY
GENERAL INFIRMARY
GREAT GEORGE STREET,
LEEDS LS1 3EX;

D1420848

# Pocket Picture Guides

# Medical Mycology

**Yvonne Clayton** BSc, PhD

Senior Lecturer
The Institute of Dermatology
St. John's Hospital for Diseases of the Skin
London, UK

**Gillian Midgley** BSc

Lecturer
The Institute of Dermatology
St. John's Hospital for Diseases of the Skin
London, UK

Gower Medical Publishing · London · New York · 1985

© Copyright 1985 by Gower Medical Publishing Ltd.
34-42 Cleveland Street, London W1P 5FB, England.

Distribution limited to United Kingdom


ISBN 0-906923-56-5


Clayton, Yvonne
  Medical mycology. –
  (Pocket picture guides to clinical medicine; 7)
  1. Fungi, Pathogenic
  I. Title   II. Midgley, Gillian   III. Series
  616'.015   QR245


Project Editor: Fiona Carr
      Designer: Eva Bozser


Printed in Italy by Imago Publishing Ltd.

# Contents

# INTRODUCTION

Fungi are a large, diverse group of organisms, sufficiently different from other living matter to be considered as a separate kingdom. They are eukaryotic, possessing a nucleus with a nuclear membrane and have a cell wall consisting of polysaccharides, polypeptides and chitin. They show heterotropic nutrition and must live as saprophytes, parasites or commensals on or in an organic substrate. Their growth form may be unicellular, as in the **yeasts**, or multicellular when the cells elongate to form filaments, known as **hyphae**, which produce a network of **mycelium**, as in the **moulds**.

Propagation in fungi is achieved by the formation of specialized cells, **spores** and **conidia**. **Spores** are produced either sexually, after fusion of nuclei followed by meiosis, or asexually by the cleavage of cell contents in a sporangium. **Conidia** are formed directly from the hyphae either by differentiation of hyphal cells as in **arthroconidia** (**arthrospores**) and **chlamydoconidia** (**chlamydospores**) or by budding from the hyphal tip or wall when they may be unicellular, **microconidia**, or multicellular, **macroconidia**.

The presence of sexual spores, zygospores, ascospores or basidiospores determines the taxonomic grouping of fungi as Zygomycota, Ascomycota or Basidiomycota. Another major group, the Deuteromycota or Fungi Imperfecti, essentially consists of Ascomycota which have lost the sexual or perfect phase in the life cycle and therefore reproduce solely by the production of conidia. Many medically important fungi are represented here and even those which do have a sexual phase are usually identified from their conidial state, as it is this form which is encountered in the laboratory.

The yeasts are a heterogeneous collection of fungi where the dominant vegetative phase is unicellular. They have members in more than one of the major taxonomic groups but characteristically they reproduce by budding, where daughter cell, **blastoconidium** (**blastospore**) is formed at the surface of the parent cell.

iv

In precise mycological terminology, the word spore is
sed only in the circumstances described above, however,
 this book, it has been retained as a general term for
 productive cells.

In fungal infections of man and animals both yeasts and
yphae may invade the tissues and the morphology of a
ngus during its existence as a parasite may differ
arkedly from its form when isolated in culture. For
ample, dermatophytes when invading the dead keratin
 skin or hair are only able to produce hyphae and
throspores. Once cultured on a suitable medium, other
atures, such as conidia, are produced by which the
ngus can be identified. Dimorphic fungi (for example,
*istoplasma capsulatum*) have a filamentous phase when
prophytic and grown in the laboratory at 26°C.
owever, when the conidia produced by this phase enter
suitable host, they are converted to yeast cells which are
ore readily disseminated in the tissues, and these may
 demonstrated by incubating cultures at 37°C.

The variety of fungi pathogenic for man and animals
ll be illustrated in the following sections according to
e infections they produce.

Details of the original descriptions of the species of
ngi, of their life cycles and taxonomy are beyond the
ope of this book, as also would be full information on
e epidemiology, clinical presentation, prognosis and
erapy of the diseases they cause. Further reading on
ese aspects is therefore suggested on page 83.

## knowledgements

e authors would like to thank the following for the use
their photographs: Miss D. Coombs, Brompton
spital (Figs.131, 134); Miss M.K. Moore, Institute of
rmatology (Figs. 70, 86, 91-95); the late Dr. R.W.
ldell (Figs.24, 160-162); Dr. D. Vella Briffa, Malta
g.120).

other illustrations are the copyright of the Institute of
rmatology.

# SUPERFICIAL MYCOSES

## Dermatophytoses

Dermatophytes are a group of closely related fungi with the ability to colonize keratinized tissues. They are identified according to the features produced when grown on a suitable agar medium and the classification into three genera is based on the shape of the macroconidia:-

1. Epidermophyton - pyriform, rough walls
2. Trichophyton - cylindrical, smooth walls
3. Microsporum - fusiform, rough walls

Dermatophytes may be described as anthropophilic, zoophilic or geophilic depending upon whether their normal habitat is on man, on an animal or in the soil.

| Anthropophilic species | Zoophilic species | Geophilic species |
|---|---|---|
| Epidermophyton floccosum | T. mentagrophytes | M. gypseum |
| Trichophyton interdigitale | T. erinacei | |
| T. rubrum | T. verrucosum | |
| T. tonsurans | T. equinum | |
| T. violaceum | T. gallinae | |
| T. soudanense | T. quinckeanum | |
| T. schoenleinii | T. simii | |
| T. concentricum | | |
| T. megninii | M. canis | |
| T. gourvilii | M. persicolor | |
| T. yaoundei | M. equinum | |
| Microsporum audouinii | M. nanum | |
| M. ferrugineum | | |
| M. rivalieri | | |

The anthropophilic species are the most successful parasites among the dermatophytes because of their ability to grow and persist in keratin with minimal excitation of the host's immune response.

The zoophilic and geophilic species tend to produce more inflammatory infections in man which may clear spontaneously.

Dermatophytes or 'ringworm' infections are often described using the Latin term 'Tinea', followed by the Latin name of the site, e.g. scalp ringworm = Tinea capitis.

# Anthropophilic species

## Epidermophyton floccosum

This is a common cause of groin and foot infections, and occasionally also body and nail infections. Hairs are not infected.

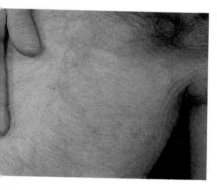

**Fig.1** Tinea cruris.

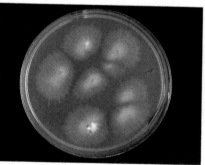

**Fig.2** Fast-growing flat colonies at 10 days with a powdery surface. The colour is olive green or khaki and, with age, radiating furrows develop. Tufts of white floccose growth appear on the surface.

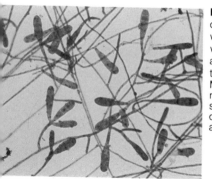

**Fig.3** Pyriform macro-conidia are numerous with slightly rough walls; their appearance is diagnostic of the species. Microconidia are never formed. Hyphal swellings and chlamydospores are common. *(x128)*

## *Trichophyton interdigitale*

This may cause foot and groin infection; it is responsible for the inflammatory type of athlete's foot which may have an associated id eruption.

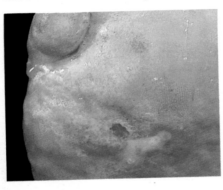

**Fig.4** Tinea pedis showing blisters.

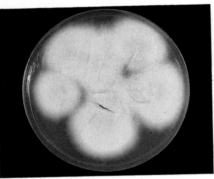

**Fig.5** Colonies at 1 days; they are white and floccose at first, becoming powdery and cream in the centre as spores develop.

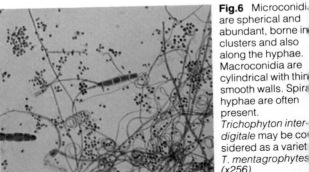

**Fig.6** Microconidia are spherical and abundant, borne in clusters and also along the hyphae. Macroconidia are cylindrical with thin smooth walls. Spiral hyphae are often present.
*Trichophyton interdigitale* may be considered as a variety *T. mentagrophytes* (x256)

3

### *Trichophyton rubrum*

*Trichophyton rubrum* causes groin, foot and nail infections; it can also cause body and facial lesions. Infections tend to become chronic and may be wide-spread. It is the main cause of destructive nail infections.

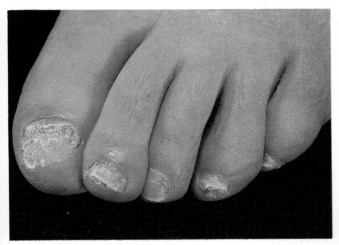

**Fig.7** Tinea unguium.

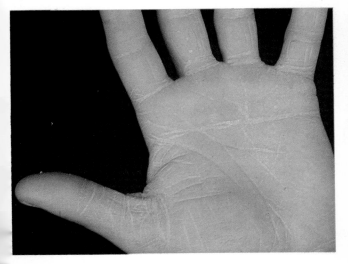

**Fig.8** Tinea manuum

The morphology of *Trichophyton rubrum* colonies is variable. All colonies (Figs. 9-11) are at 14 days.

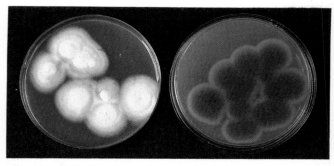

**Fig.9** Most frequently cultures are white and floccose with red to brown pigment on the reverse side.

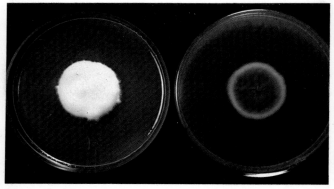

**Fig.10** Some isolates produce a melanoid pigment which diffuses into the medium and colours the entire plate.

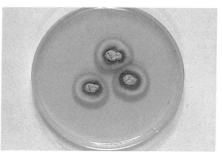

**Fig.11** Granular variety.

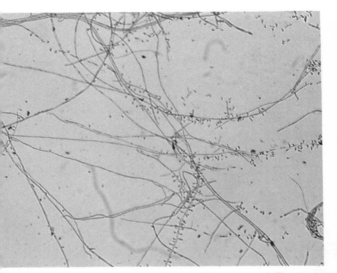

**Fig.12** Microconidia are numerous or scanty (2-3 x 3-5μ). They are oval, slender and borne along the sides of hyphae. *(x192)*

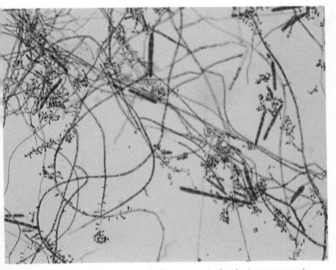

**Fig.13** Macroconidia are rare in floccose strains but numerous in granular colonies. They are long, cylindrical and have thin, smooth walls. *(x384)*

## *Trichophyton tonsurans*

*Trichophyton tonsurans* is a cause of endothrix scalp infection, which does not fluoresce; it also causes skin and nail infections.

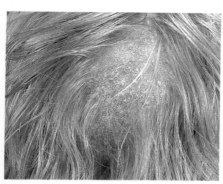

**Fig.14** Tinea capitis.

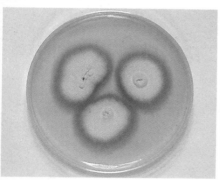

**Fig.15** Colonies at 14 days. They are initially white on the surface but with the production of spores become grey or yellow and powdery in texture. The centre of the colony becomes folded and a crater may be formed. Brown pigment is seen on the reverse side.

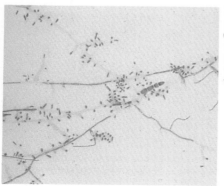

**Fig.16** Microconidia are numerous, large (3-5 x 9-7μ) and borne along the sides of hyphae. Chlamydospores are frequent. *(x256)*

## Trichophyton violaceum

This occurs most commonly in the Middle East, Mediterranean countries, parts of Africa, India and Asia. It causes endothrix scalp infection and also affects skin and nails.

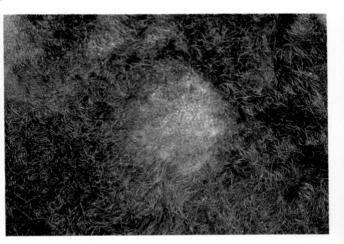

**Fig.17** Tinea capitis.

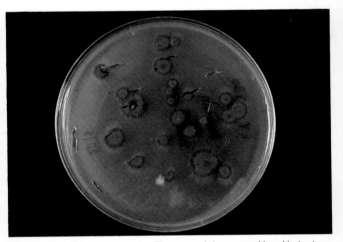

**Fig.18** Colonies at two weeks. They are glabrous and hard in texture with restricted growth. The colour is dark red or purple.
Microscopical examination shows numerous hyphal swellings and chlamydospores; microconidia and macroconidia are rare or absent.

## *Trichophyton soudanense*

There is widespread distribution in Africa, but *Trichophyton soudanense* has also recently been isolated from several other areas. It causes endothrix scalp infection and also affects the skin and nails.

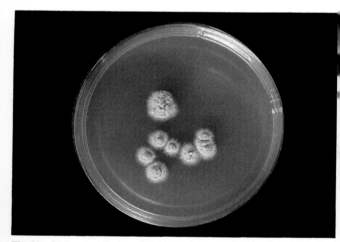

**Fig.19** Glabrous colonies at 20 days with a finely folded surface and stellate fringe. The texture is like suede and the colour is usually yellow or orange, but some isolates eventually deepen to dark red.

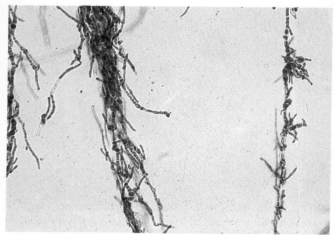

**Fig.20** The mycelium is characterized by the division of some hyphae into short, angular segments with reflexive branches. *(x384)*

### *Trichophyton schoenleinii*

*Trichophyton schoenleinii* occurs mainly in parts of the Middle East and North Africa. It is a cause of favus, a chronic disease of the scalp distinguished by the formation of crusts (scutula), permanent hair loss and scarring. The infection is endothrix, often of long lengths of hair which fluoresce dull green. The characteristic feature is the presence of air spaces in the hair (Fig.177). Both adults and children are affected; skin lesions also occur.

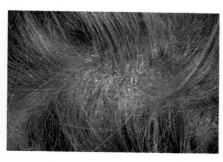

**Fig.21**  Favus of scalp.

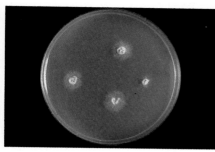

**Fig.22**  Slow growing, glabrous and compact colonies at 21 days. The colour is white or grey, the surface convoluted and there is considerable submerged growth.

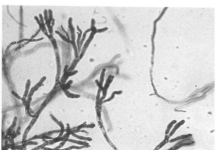

**Fig.23**  The characteristic feature is the presence of 'antler' hyphae. Hyphal swellings and chlamydospores are frequent. Microconidia and macroconidia are absent. *(x256)*

## Trichophyton concentricum

*Trichophyton concentricum* is found mainly in the South Pacific. It is the causative organism of tinea imbricata.

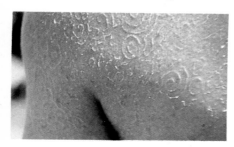

**Fig.24** Tinea imbricata.

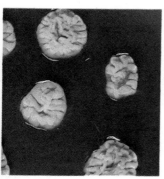

**Fig.25** Slow growing and glabrous colonies at 21 days, which are soft in texture. The surface is raised and the colour grey or buff. Microscopical examination shows hyphal swellings and numerous chlamydospores. Microconidia and macroconidia are rare.

## Trichophyton megninii

*Trichophyton megninii* occurs in Europe, particularly Portugal and Sardinia. It is the cause of body, foot and nail ringworm and also infects beard and scalp hairs with an ectothrix infection which does not fluoresce.

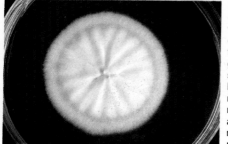

**Fig.26** Colony at 14 days. The surface is white and fluffy, developing a pink tinge and radial grooves. The reverse shows a red pigment. Microscopical examination shows clavate microconidia borne along the hyphae; macroconidia are rare.

## *Trichophyton gourvilii*

*Trichophyton gourvilii* is found only in parts of Africa where it causes endothrix scalp infection; skin and nail infections also occur.

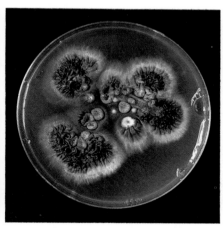

**Fig.27** Colonies at 21 days are folded and raised in the centre with a soft glabrous texture. The surface is red or purple often with a white border. Microscopical examination shows oval microconidia borne along the hyphae; macroconidia are rare.

## *Trichophyton yaoundei*

*Trichophyton yaoundei* is found in Equatorial Africa where it causes endothrix scalp infection.

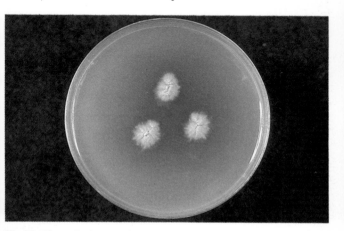

**Fig.28** The colonies are slow-growing and glabrous in texture at 21 days; they are white at first but become brown or tan with age. Microscopical examination rarely shows either microconidia or macroconidia.

## *Microsporum audouinii*

*Microsporum audouinii* causes tinea capitis and is responsible for the classical epidemic form, although infections by this species are now rare in Europe. Hairs show a small-spored ectothrix infection.

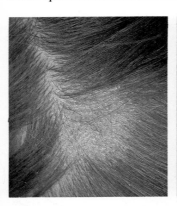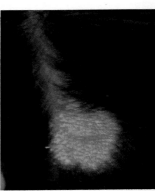

**Fig.29** Tinea capitis and fluorescence under Wood's lamp.

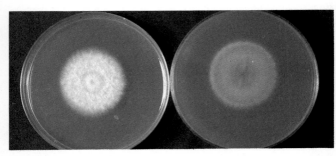

**Fig.30** The colony at 14 days shows sparse white surface growth with a salmon pink to brown colour on the reverse.

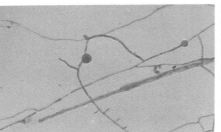

**Fig.31** Microconidia are long, clavate and borne along hyphae; they may be scanty. Macroconidia are rare; and are often distorted in shape. Chlamydospores are present. *(x256)*

# Microsporum ferrugineum

*Microsporum ferrugineum* is a common cause of scalp
infection in Asia, Africa, USSR and Eastern Europe; it is
uncommon in the West.

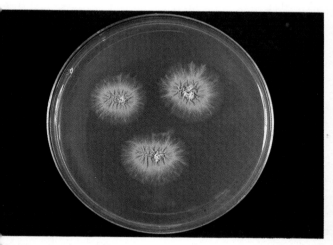

**Fig.32** Folded, leathery colonies at 21 days which are rust or fawn in
colour.

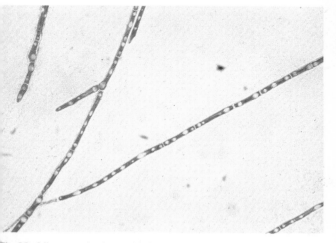

**Fig.33** Microscopical examination shows thick-walled hyphae with
prominent cross walls but otherwise no characteristic features.
Microconidia are rare; macroconidia are absent. *(x384)*

14

### *Microsporum rivalieri*
This is a cause of scalp infection in Africa.

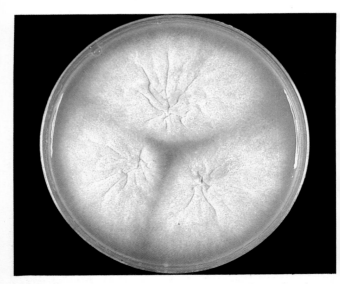

**Fig.34** Colonies at 21 days are white and folded. The surface has a satin sheen or the appearance of ground-glass.

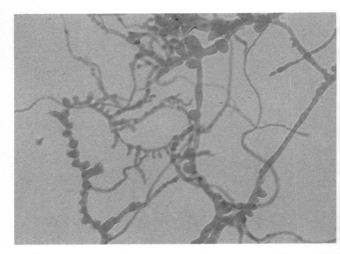

**Fig.35** Numerous pectinate hyphae are characteristic. Microconidia and macroconidia are absent. *(x384)*

# Zoophilic species

## *Trichophyton mentagrophytes*

*Trichophyton mentagrophytes* is a cause of small-spored, non-fluorescent ectothrix infection in domestic, farm and laboratory animals and a wide variety of wild animals. It also causes human infections of the scalp, beard and skin.

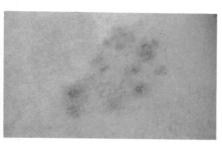

**Fig.36** Tinea corporis.

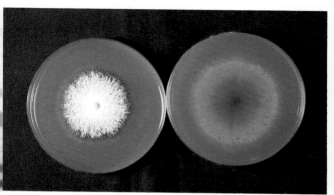

**Fig.37** Colony at 14 days. There is a powdery or granular surface, white or cream in colour, often with a radiate margin. A dark brown or red pigment often develops on the reverse.

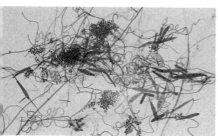

**Fig.38** Microconidia are numerous, spherical and borne in clusters as well as along the hyphae. Macroconidia are cylindrical and thin-walled. Spiral hyphae are often present. *(x128)*

### *Trichophyton erinacei*

*Trichophyton erinacei* is a specific cause of hedgehog infections in Britain and New Zealand. It causes body lesions in humans and occasional ectothrix hair infection. The hairs do not fluoresce.

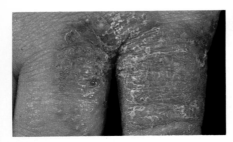

**Fig.39** Tinea manuum

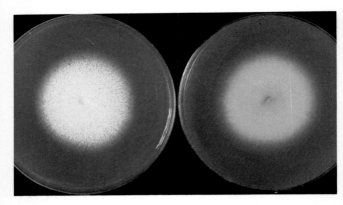

**Fig.40** The colony at 14 days has a flat surface and is powdery and white in colour. Yellow pigment is produced on the reverse of the colony.

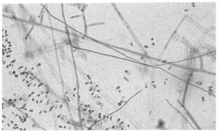

**Fig.41** Microconidia are numerous, elongated in shape and borne along the hyphae. Macroconidia are cylindrical and thin-walled. Spiral hyphae may be present. *(x256)*

17

## *Trichophyton verrucosum*

*Trichophyton verrucosum* causes large-spored ectothrix infection in cattle and man; infected hairs do not fluoresce. Human beard and body lesions may be severe and inflammatory.

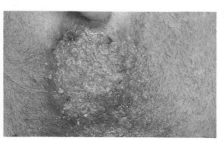

**Fig.42** Tinea barbae.

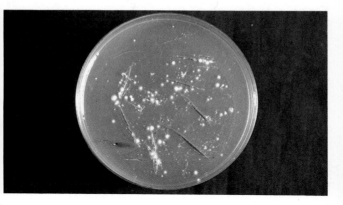

**Fig.43** Colonies at 14 days. They are slow-growing with a glabrous, hard texture and are white or buff in colour. Growth is faster at 37°C than at 26°C.

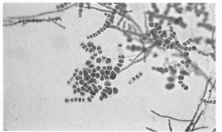

**Fig.44** Hyphal swellings and chlamydospores are present. Microconidia and macroconidia are absent. *(x256)*

## *Trichophyton equinum*

This is a cause of ectothrix infection in horses and rarely of body infection in man.

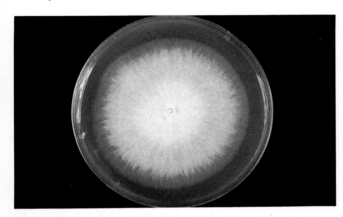

**Fig.45** Colony at 21 days. There is a white surface with a velvety texture which becomes buff or pink with age. The reverse is yellow in young colonies but brown pigment rapidly develops.
Microscopical examination shows spherical or oval microconidia borne along the hyphae. Macroconidia are cylindrical and thin-walled. Spiral hyphae may be present.

## *Trichophyton gallinae*

This is a cause of infection in chickens and other fowl; it rarely causes disease in man.

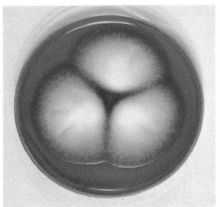

**Fig.46** Colonies are white and flat with a cottony texture at 21 days. Strawberry red pigment is present on the reverse which diffuses throughout the medium. Microscopical examination shows clavate microconidia borne along the hyphae. Macroconidia are spoon-shaped when present.

## *Trichophyton quinckeanum*

This is a cause of mouse favus; infections are rare in man.

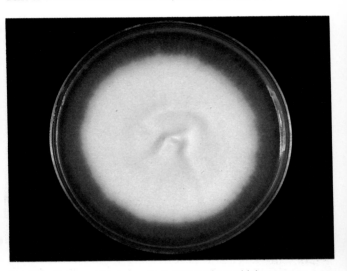

**Fig.47a** Colony at 21 days with a white surface which appears smooth and cottony; folds and a central crater are formed with age. The culture has a characteristic sour odour.

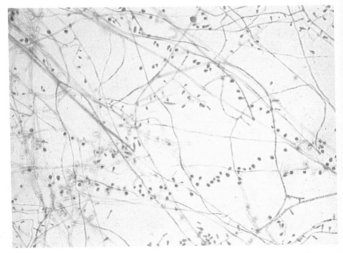

**b** Microscopical examination shows oval microconidia borne along the hyphae. Macroconidia are rarely present. (x384)

## Trichophyton simii

*Trichophyton simii* is a cause of infection of monkeys and chickens in India. It can produce inflammatory infection in man. There is a large-spored ectothrix infection in animal hairs with green fluorescence.

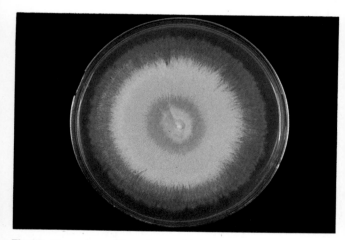

**Fig.48** The surface of the colony at 21 days is powdery and buff or pink in colour. The reverse is yellow, buff or red.

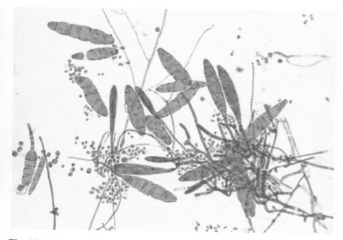

**Fig.49** Microconidia are elongated and pear-shaped. Macroconidia are numerous and elongated with smooth, thin walls and with characteristic swollen segments. *(x384)*

### *Microsporum canis*

*Microsporum canis* causes infection in kittens and puppies which may be transmitted to man giving rise to scalp and body lesions. Hairs show a small-spored ecto-thrix infection with bright green fluorescence.

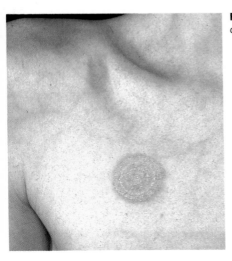

**Fig.50** Tinea corporis.

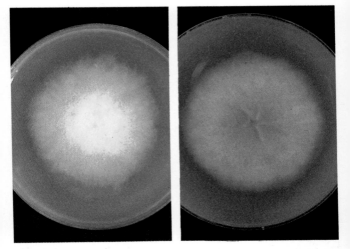

**Fig.51** A colony at 14 days shows abundant white aerial mycelium becoming buff in colour; bright yellow or orange pigment is present on the reverse.

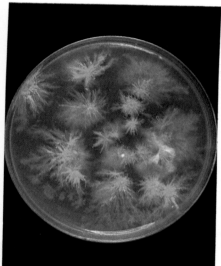

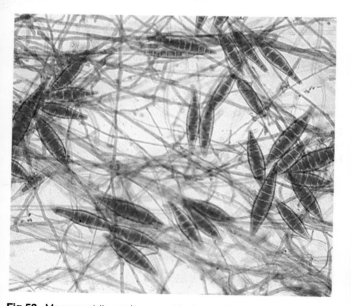

**Fig.53** Macroconidia are large and fusiform with thick, rough walls and are diagnostic of the species. *(x192)*

23

### *Microsporum persicolor*

*Microsporum persicolor* is associated with small mammals, especially voles, in Europe and USA. It is an uncommon cause of infection in man.

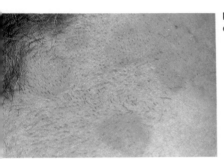

**Fig.54** Tinea corporis.

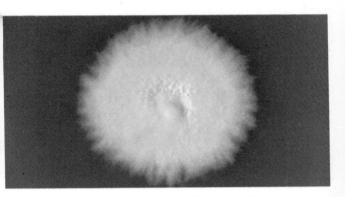

**Fig.55** Colony at 14 days. There is a fluffy and powdery texture, often with a fringed margin; the surface and reverse are cream or pink.

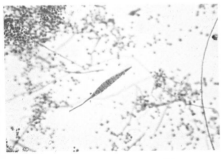

**Fig.56** Microconidia are numerous and clavate. Macroconidia are narrow, clavate and thin-walled. *(x128)*

### *Microsporum equinum*

*Microsporum equinum* is primarily a pathogen of horses, and is rarely transmitted to man.

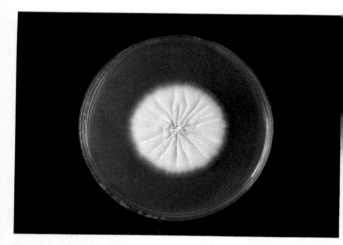

**Fig.57**  A colony at 14 days with thin, white surface growth and a velvety texture with radial grooves. Cream or pink pigment is present on the reverse.

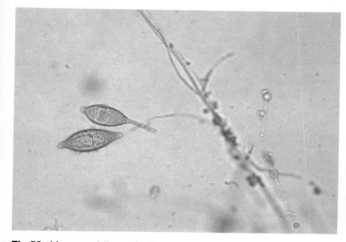

**Fig.58**  Macroconidia are fusiform and thick-walled but shorter and fatter than those of *M. canis*; this appearance is diagnostic of the species. *(x384)*

# *Microsporum nanum*

*Microsporum nanum* is primarily a cause of infection in pigs in Europe, Asia and America; it is a rare cause of scalp and body infections in man.

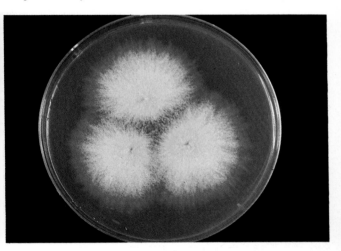

**Fig.59** Flat colonies at 14 days with a powdery buff surface; the reverse often appears red to brown.

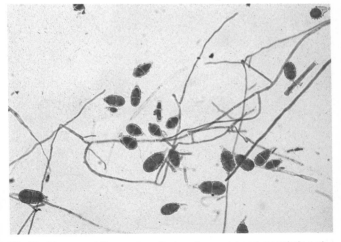

**Fig.60** Macroconidia are abundant and egg-shaped, consisting of only one to three cells with rough walls. *(x192)*

# Geophilic species

## *Microsporum gypseum*

*Microsporum gypseum* is found world-wide in the soil but is an uncommon cause of scalp and body infections in man

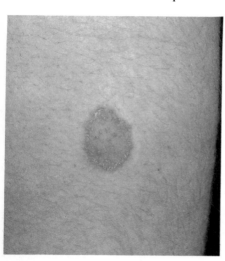

**Fig.61** Tinea corporis.

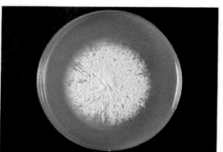

**Fig.62** Powdery and buff to cinnamon coloured colony at 10 days.

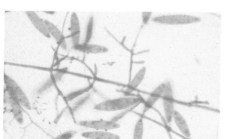

**Fig.63** Microconidia are abundant and clavate. Macroconidia are numerous, oval or boat-shaped with thin, rough walls diagnostic of the species. *(x256)*

# Other superficial mycoses

| Disease | Causative fungus |
|---|---|
| Pityriasis versicolor | *Malassezia furfur* |
| Tinea nigra | *Exophiala werneckii* |
| Black piedra | *Piedraia hortae* |
| White piedra | *Trichosporon beigelii* |
| Otomycosis | *Aspergillus niger* <br> *A. fumigatus*, other <br> *Aspergilli, Mucor* <br> species and yeasts |
| Mycotic keratitis | *Aspergillus* species <br> *Fusarium* species <br> *Candida* species, etc. |
| Onychomycosis | *Scopulariopsis brevicaulis* <br> *Acremonium* species, etc. |
| *Hendersonula* infections | *Hendersonula toruloidea* |
| *Scytalidium* infections | *Scytalidium hyalinum* |
| Candidosis | *Candida albicans* <br> other *Candida* species. |

# Pityriasis versicolor

**Causative fungus**: *Malassezia furfur*

This infection has a world-wide distribution but is most prevalent in the tropics. It is characterized by the development of brown-coloured scaly macules which most frequently occur on the chest, back or upper arms. Hypopigmented lesions may appear on exposed areas which have been suntanned. Lesions sometimes fluoresce a golden colour under Wood's lamp.

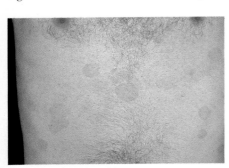

**Fig.64** Hyper-pigmented lesions.

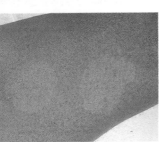

**Fig.65** Hypopigmented lesions.

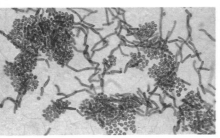

**Fig.66** Infected skin scales in Parker's stain showing thick-walled yeasts, 3-8μ in diameter, and short angular hyphae. *(x256)*

Culture is of no value for diagnostic purposes since the yeasts alone may be present as skin commensals.

# Tinea nigra

**Causative fungus:** *Exophiala werneckii*
This infection has been reported most frequently in
Central and South America and the Caribbean.

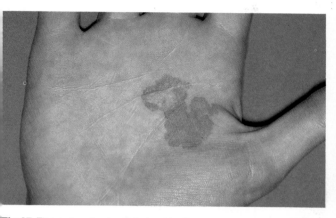

**Fig.67** Tinea nigra is characterized by the appearance of smooth,
brown lesions which are usually on the palms, but occasionally on the
feet.

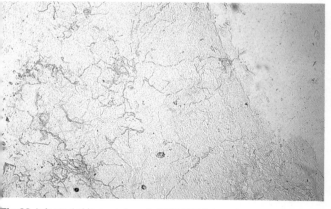

**Fig.68** Infected skin scrapings in 30% KOH show brown, septate,
irregularly branched hyphae, 2-5μ in diameter. *(x96)*

Colonies are initially pale and moist, consisting of
yeasts, some with septa, but older cultures become dark
green or black with pigmented hyphae producing numerous conidia.

# Black piedra

### Causative fungus: *Piedraia hortae*

Black piedra is an infection most commonly reported from humid and tropical countries, particularly in Central and South America, where dark, gritty nodules appear on the shafts of scalp hairs.

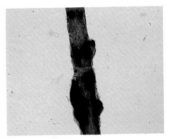

**Fig.69** Hair in 30% KOH showing dark nodules, initially formed under the cuticle. The nodules consist of regularly arranged, thick-walled cells and hyphae held together by a cement-like substance. *(x64)*

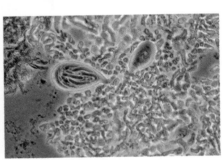

**Fig.70** Larger nodules may contain asci with distinctive fusiform ascospores. *(Phase contrast, x300)*

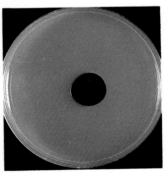

**Fig.71** Slow-growing dark brown or black colonies at 26°C.

Microscopical examination shows dark, thick-walled, closely septate hyphae with intercalary chlamydospores. Asci are rarely produced in culture.

31

# White piedra

**Causative fungus**: *Trichosporon beigelii*

White piedra is an infection of beard, axillary or pubic hairs which have pale, soft nodules that may coalesce. It occurs in temperate regions of the Orient, South America, USA and Europe.

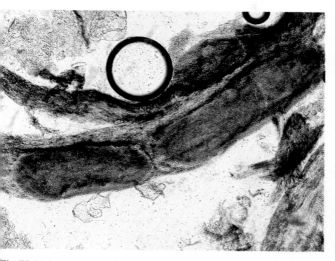

**Fig.72** Hair showing white nodules consisting of hyaline hyphae and arthrospores which readily take up Parker's stain. *(x96)*

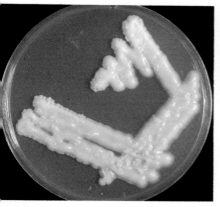

**Fig.73** Colonies at 5 days at 37°C on Sabouraud dextrose agar without cyclo-heximide. The texture may be soft and mucoid or tough and fibrous with a wrinkled surface.

Microscopical examination shows yeasts, hyphae and arthrospores.

# Otomycosis

**Causative fungi**: *Aspergillus niger*, *A. fumigatus*, **other** *Aspergilli*, *Mucor* **species and yeasts.**
This is a superficial, chronic or subacute infection of the outer ear canal, characterized by inflammation, scaling, pruritus and pain. Fungi are often superimposed on a bacterial infection.

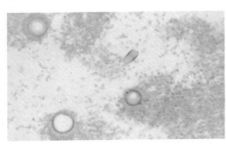

**Fig.74** Section of exudate showing sporing heads of *Aspergillus niger*. *(x128)*

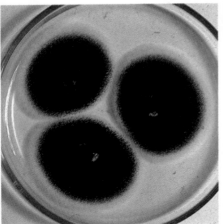

**Fig.75** Colonies of *Aspergillus niger* grown at 37°C.

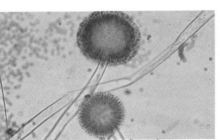

**Fig.76** Sporing heads of *Aspergillus niger*. *(x128)*

# Mycotic keratitis

**Causative fungi**: **Aspergilli (mainly *Aspergillus fumigatus*); *Fusarium* species (especially *Fusarium solani*); *Candida* species and many other fungi.**
This is an infection on the surface of the cornea which usually follows an injury to the eye. Corneal ulcers caused by fungi may be of any shape or type depending on which species is involved.

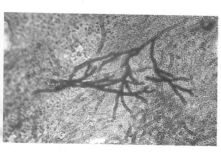

**Fig.77** Scraping from corneal ulcer showing hyphae. *(x256)*

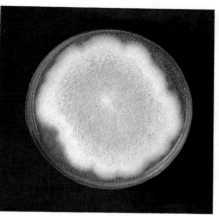

**Fig.78** *Fusarium solani* culture.

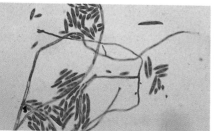

**Fig.79** Hyaline macroconidia of *F. solani* which are two to several celled and cylindrical to curved in shape with a distinctive foot cell. (x256).

# Onychomycosis

A variety of filamentous non-dermatophytes may cause nail infections, particularly after damage to the nail by trauma or disease. Toenails, especially hallux nails, are affected more frequently than fingernails.

**Causative fungi:** *Scopulariopsis brevicaulis*; *Acremonium* species; *Aspergillus* species; *Fusarium* species.

Many of these fungi are common in the environment and it is, therefore, necessary that their isolation from nails should be confirmed whenever possible by repeated isolations. Confirmatory evidence of the significance of an isolation may sometimes be obtained from the clinical appearance of the nail and the morphology of the fungus seen on microscopy. Two examples are: *Scopulariopsis brevicaulis* infection and superficial white onychomycosis.

### *Scopulariopsis brevicaulis* infection

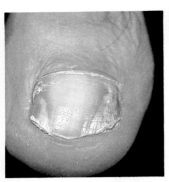

**Fig.80** Infected nail showing typical brown discoloration with crumbling of the nailplate.

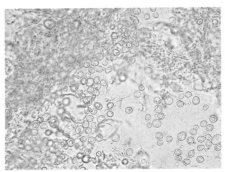

**Fig.81** Nail in 30% KOH showing thick-walled, lemon-shaped spores and scanty hyphae. *(x256)*

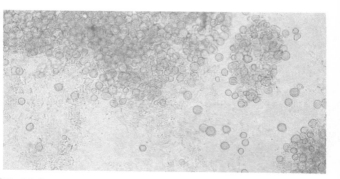

**Fig.82** Spores in nails readily take up Parker's stain. *(x320)*

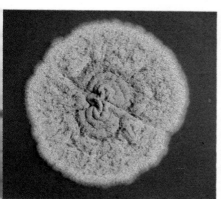

**Fig.83** White waxy colony with cerebriform folding, which becomes brown and powdery as it ages on a medium without cycloheximide.

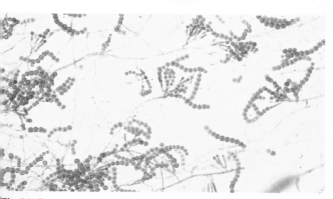

**Fig.84** Chains of rough, thick-walled lemon-shaped spores. *(x160)*

# Superficial white onychomycosis

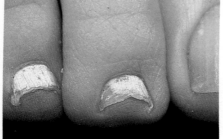

**Fig.85** Crumbly white patches are present on the surface of the nail. The infection is very superficial and material may be collected by scraping the nail surface with a scalpel.

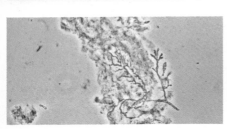

**Fig.86** *Acremonium* species in nail in 30% KOH, showing characteristic fronding hyphae. *(Phase contrast, x120)*

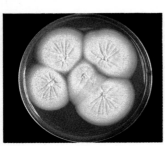

**Fig.87** White to pale pink wrinkled colonies of *Acremonium* species.

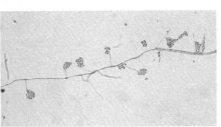

**Fig.88** Tapering phialides arise from vegetative hyphae; conidia typically occur in balls at the apices of phialides. *(x96)*

The dermatophyte, *Trichophyton interdigitale*, may also produce this condition of the nails.

# *Hendersonula toruloidea* infection

*Hendersonula toruloidea* is a filamentous non-dermatophyte which may cause a chronic infection of the soles, palms and nails, which is clinically indistinguishable from *Trichophyton rubrum* infection. Infections occur in patients from the tropics, particularly the Caribbean, Africa and the Indian sub-continent.

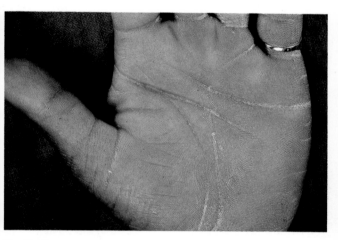

**Fig.89** Chronic infection of the palm.

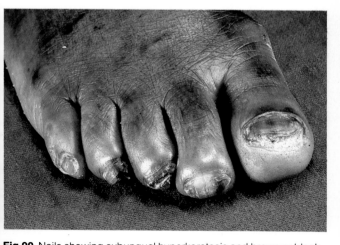

**Fig.90** Nails showing subungual hyperkeratosis and brown or black discoloration.

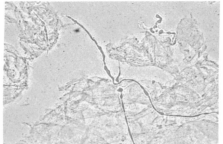

**Fig.91** Scrapings in 30% KOH which resemble those of a dermatophyte but show more variation in width along their length and a double-contoured appearance due to retraction of the cytoplasm from the hyphal cell wall. *(Phase contrast, x300)*

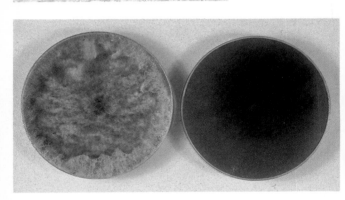

**Fig.92** Fast-growing colony form on Sabouraud dextrose agar without cycloheximide after 3-4 days at 26°C with high, cottony, aerial mycelium, initially white, but darkening to grey or black as it ages.

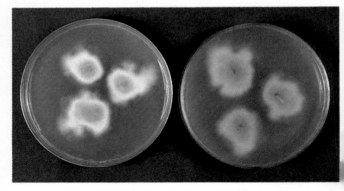

**Fig.93** Slowly-growing form (10-14 days) with velvety or 'wire-wool' texture and grey-brown colour.

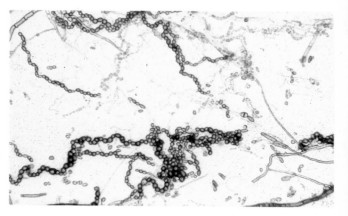

**Fig.94** Chains of one to two-celled arthrospores, initially hyaline but later brown; rough-walled hyphae and large hyphal coils may also be present. *(x192)*

## *Scytalidium hyalinum* infection

*Scytalidium hyalinum* is a non-dermatophyte producing infections closely resembling those of *H. toruloidea*. The fungus has so far only been isolated from patients of West Indian, Guyanan and West African origin.

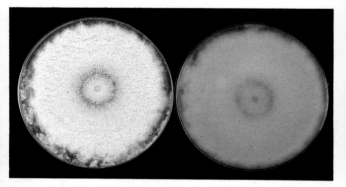

**Fig.95** Fast-growing colony with fairly high aerial mycelium, which is white or buff-cream in colour.

Microscopical examination shows chains of irregularly-shaped hyaline arthrospores.

# Candidosis

**Causative organism**: *Candida albicans*; occasionally other *Candida* species.

Superficial infections caused by yeasts of the genus Candida are very common and are found in all parts of the world. They include oral and vaginal candidosis, and involvement of the skin (particularly intertriginous areas) and nails. *Candida albicans* is a commensal of the alimentary tract.

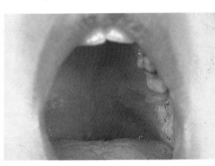

**Fig.96** Oral candidosis showing white adherent membranes on the buccal mucosa.

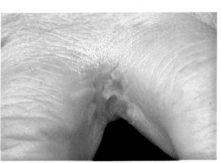

**Fig.97** Intertrigo of a finger web showing white, macerated skin.

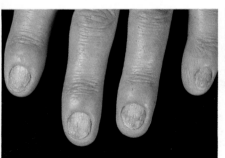

**Fig.98** Redness and swelling of finger nailfolds with distortion and discoloration of the nailplate caused by infection with *Candida albicans*.

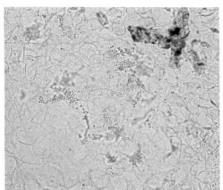

**Fig.99** Skin in 30% KOH showing hyphae and yeasts. *(x130)*

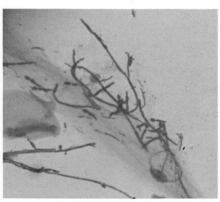

**Fig.100** Vaginal exudate showing gram stained hyphae and yeasts. *(x280)*

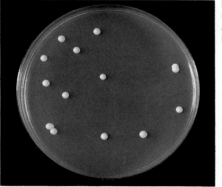

**Fig.101** Colonies of *Candida albicans* after 48 hours incubation at 37°C.

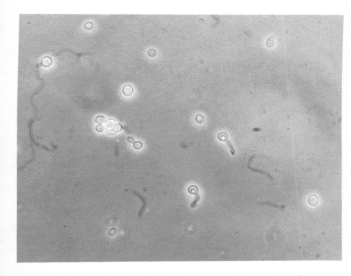

**Fig.102** Identification of *Candida albicans* can be made by the demonstration of germ tubes produced by the yeasts after 2 hours incubation in serum at 37°C. *(Phase contrast, x450)*

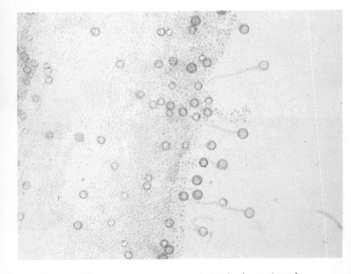

**Fig.103** Identification may also be made by the formation of chlamydospores (vesicles) on the filaments seen in Rice/Tween agar after 48 hours incubation at 26°C. *(x180)*

# SUBCUTANEOUS MYCOSES

Infections of the cutaneous and subcutaneous tissues are caused by a variety of fungi from many unrelated genera. Occasionally skin scrapings from the lesion may be sufficient to demonstrate the pathogen but biopsy specimens are usually required. Histological examination is frequently characteristic enough for a diagnosis to be made, but a culture should be performed for confirmation.

These diseases are seen mainly in tropical and subtropical parts of the world where the causative fungi are found in the soil or on plant material. Some form of trauma is necessary to introduce the fungal spores into the subepidermal tissues.

The fungi may be isolated on Sabouraud dextrose agar, but many of these pathogens are sensitive to cycloheximide and in these cases this antibiotic should be omitted from the medium. Cultures should be maintained for 3-4 weeks.

## Mycetoma

The disease presents as localized swollen lesions, usually on the foot or hand, which contain grains composed of the aetiological agent. The grains may be found in fluid from draining sinuses, and are either white, red or black and may be hard in texture due to the presence of cement. Infection results from the introduction of the causative organism into the skin and subcutaneous tissues, possibly associated with a foreign body (e.g. a thorn or splinter).

The causative agents, consisting of a variety of actinomycetes and fungi, probably live in the soil and on vegetable matter; their geographical distribution is influenced by climate, particularly the amount of rainfall.

The distinction between actinomycetoma (caused by actinomycetes) and eumycetoma (caused by fungi) is made by the size of the filaments seen on examination of the grains in wet preparation in KOH, or in section.

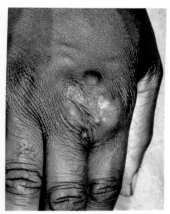

**Fig.104** Mycetoma of the hand.

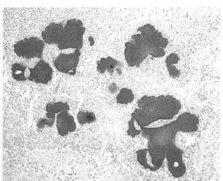

**Fig.105** Section of actinomycetoma grain (*Actinomadura pelletieri*). The filaments are about 1 micron in diameter. *(H & E, x64)*

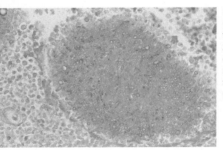

**Fig.106** Section of pale grain eumycetoma. Filaments are 2-5 microns in diameter and are septate. Chlamydospores are often present. *(PAS, x160)*

Grains should be washed thoroughly in saline solution before culture.

45

**ctinomycetoma** Causative organisms include:
 *Actinomadura madurae*
 *A. pelletieri*
 *Nocardia asteroides*
 *N. brasiliensis*
 *Streptomyces somaliensis*
 hese actinomycetes should be grown aerobically on
 ither blood agar, nutrient agar or Sabouraud dextrose
 gar without the addition of antibacterial antibiotics and
 ncubated at 30°C.

## Examples of cultures

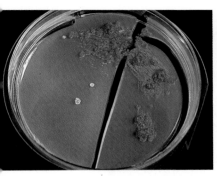

**Fig.107**
*Actinomadura pelletieri*. Colonies are waxy, wrinkled and bright red in colour.

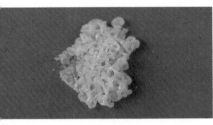

**Fig.108**
*Actinomadura madurae*. Colonies have a shiny, waxy, wrinkled surface and are white to yellow in colour.

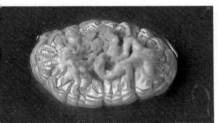

**Fig.109** *Nocardia brasiliensis*. The colony is heaped-up and folded and is white to orange in colour with a chalky surface.

Microscopical examination shows branching filaments (1 micron or less in diameter) which do not fragment.

Identification of the aerobic actinomycetes is according to the morphology of the colony and its filaments, composition of the cell wall and physiological reactions.

**Eumycetoma** Causative fungi include:
*Madurella mycetomatis*
*M. grisea*
*Pseudallescheria boydii*
*Leptospheria senagalensis*
*Acremonium, Aspergillus* and *Fusarium* species
Cultures are made on Sabouraud dextrose agar without cycloheximide, and incubated at 26°C for 3-4 weeks.

### *Examples of cultures*

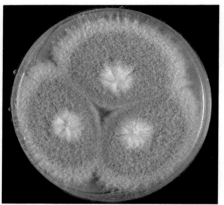

**Fig.110**
*Pseudallescheria boydii*. The colony is floccose and white at first, later becoming smoky grey in colour.

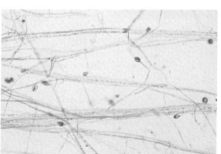

**Fig.111** Microscopical examination shows ovoid or pyriform conidia produced singly at the tips of conidiophores. (*x256*)

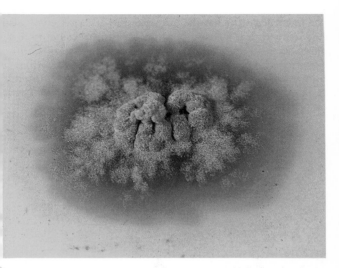

**Fig.112** *Madurella mycetomatis*. The colony is initially flat, then folded with a raised centre, varying in colour from white to brown. Most isolates produce a brown pigment that diffuses into the medium.

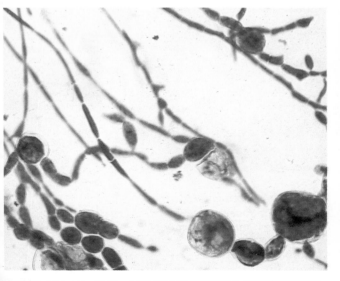

**Fig.113** Microscopical examination shows broad, irregular septate hyphae and intercalary or terminal chlamydospores. (*x384*)

48

# Chromomycosis

The disease is characterized by warty nodules, usually on the lower legs; the hands, buttocks and other sites can also be involved. It is a cosmopolitan chronic disease but most cases occur in the tropical and subtropical areas of Latin America and Africa. Infection is often associated with an injury with wood. The causative organisms are a limited group of dematiaceous fungi living saprophytically in soil on organic matter.

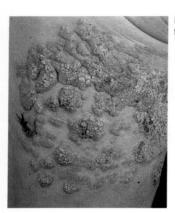

**Fig.114** Lesions on the thigh.

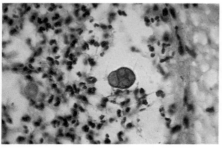

**Fig.115** In tissues, spherical, brown thick-walled fungal cells are found singly or in clusters in giant cells or within microabscesses. Cell are 5-12 microns in diameter and may be septate. (H & E,x256)

**Causative fungi** include:
*Phialophora (fonsecea) pedrosoi*
*Phialophora (fonsecea) compacta*
*Phialophora verrucosa*
*Cladosporium carrionii*
Cultures are made on Sabouraud dextrose agar and plates with antibiotics may be included. The fungi grow at 26°C and plates should be kept for up to 3 weeks.

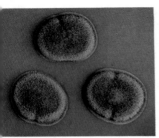

**Fig.116** Culture of *Phialophora pedrosoi*. The colony is fluffy to velvety in texture and greenish black in colour.

*Phialophora pedrosoi* is the most prevalent species and produces three types of conidiophores:

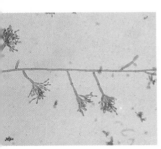

**Fig.117** *Cladosporium type* - simple conidiophore which produces chains of conidia. *(x256)*

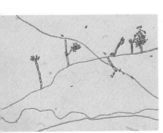

**Fig.118** *Acrotheca type* - simple conidiophore bearing oval conidia on the top and along the sides. *(x256)*

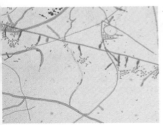

**Fig.119** *Phialophora type* - distinct flask-shaped conidiophore (phialide); conidia are formed at the end of the flask and extruded through the neck. *(x256)*

# Sporotrichosis

The disease is characterized by nodular lesions which often ulcerate. Secondary nodules may develop from the primary lesion along the course of a lymphatic. Infection results from the introduction of the fungus into the skin or subcutaneous tissues, with lesions occurring on exposed parts of the body, especially on the hands, arms or legs. The fungus occurs as a saprophyte in soil, on plants and on various plant materials.

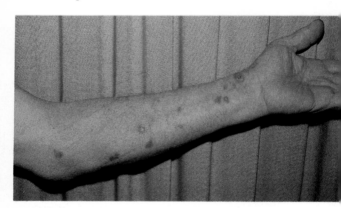

**Fig.120**   Initial lesion on the distal head of the radius.

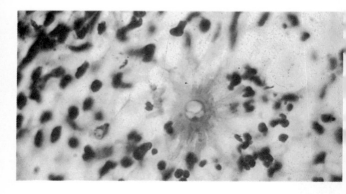

**Fig.121**   It is usually very difficult to demonstrate the causative fungus in sections or exudates from human lesions; asteroid bodies may be present - these consist of a yeast cell surrounded by stellate rays of eosinophilic substance.   *(H & E, x500)*

Cultures are necessary to confirm the diagnosis.

**Causative fungus: *Sporothrix schenckii***
This is a dimorphic fungus; it exists in a mycelial form in saprophytic life and in a yeast form in animal tissues. The mycelial form can be isolated on Sabouraud dextrose agar containing cycloheximide at 26°C, but the yeast phase is best isolated on brain/heart infusion agar at 37°C. Demonstration of the yeast form is essential to confirm identification.

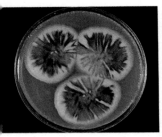

**Fig.122** Culture at 26°C (mycelial form). Small white waxy colonies appear first and later become wrinkled, membranous and the colour varies between cream and black.

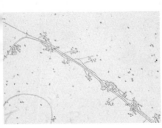

**Fig.123** Microscopical examination shows delicate mycelium bearing pear-shaped conidia which arise in clusters from the tips of hyphae and also laterally in sheaths surrounding the hyphae. (*x256*)

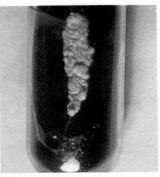

**Fig.124** Culture at 37°C (yeast form). Wrinkled, moist cream-coloured colonies are grown.

Microscopical examination shows elongated yeasts, 3 to 5 microns long.

# Zygomycosis (Phycomycosis)

## a) Basidiobolomycosis

The disease presents mostly in children as a subcutaneous swelling on the arms or legs. It has a firm consistency and does not ulcerate. The mode of infection is unknown. The disease is widely distributed in tropical and subtropical zones, particularly in East and West Africa, Indonesia and the Indian subcontinent. The fungus is found associated with decaying vegetable matter. It also occurs in the intestinal tract of frogs, toads and lizards: it is readily found growing on the dung of these animals, the spores being actively discharged.

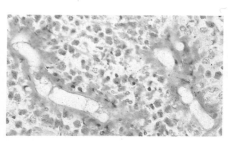

**Fig.125** Section showing wide hyphae; many are surrounded by granular eosinophilic material. (*H & E*, x256)

## Causative fungus: *Basidiobolus haptosporus*

Cultures must be made on Sabouraud dextrose agar without cycloheximide and grow better at 37°C. Colonies appear within a week.

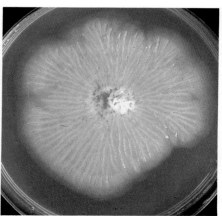

**Fig.126** The colonies are grey or tan in colour, glabrous, thin and radially folded.

Two types of spore are produced: sporangia and zygospores.

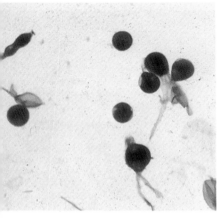

**Fig.127** Sporangia are formed at the tips of sporangiophores from which they are actively discharged by a projectile mechanism. *(x192)*

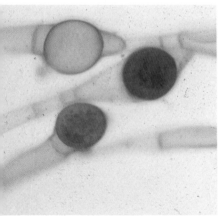

**Fig.128** Zygospores produced by the fusion of hyphae are spherical, thick-walled with a beak formed from a hyphal remnant. *(x364)*

## b) Rhinoentomophthoromycosis

Infection is limited to nasal mucosa, nasal sinuses and subcutaneous tissues of the nose and face. The fungus occurs in the soil on decaying vegetation. The disease occurs most frequently in Africa, particularly in Nigeria; other cases are reported from the Caribbean and South America.

## Causative fungus: *Conidiobolus coronatus*

Cultures must be made on Sabouraud dextrose agar without cycloheximide at 37°C.

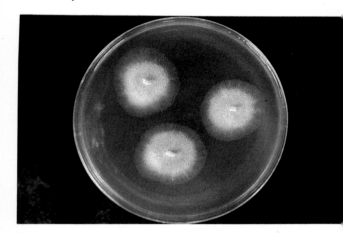

**Fig.129** Rapidly growing colonies are initially flat, adherent and glabrous, later developing radial folds and becoming velvety as aerial mycelium develops.

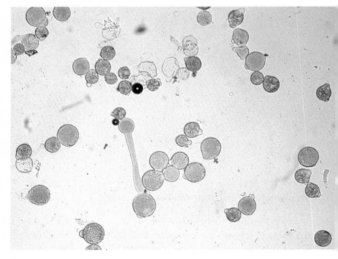

**Fig.130** Microscopical examination showing conidia which are forcibly discharged from the tips of the conidiophores. Conidia may develop hair-like appendages. *(x192)*

# SYSTEMIC MYCOSES

These diseases usually result from the inhalation of fungus-infected dust and the primary site of infection is almost always the lungs. Dissemination to any organ may occur. Most of the causative organisms have been isolated from the soil where, under suitable climatic conditions, they produce hyphae and spores. Some require such specific conditions in nature that their geographical distribution is limited (e.g. *Coccidioides immitis*) whilst others occur throughout the world (e.g. *Cryptococcus neoformans*).

Many of these fungi are dimorphic and to isolate both phases, cultures should be prepared at 26°C on Sabouraud dextrose agar with cycloheximide and at 37°C on brain/heart infusion agar. Cycloheximide should be omitted from culture medium when growing *Aspergilli*, *Candida* species, *Cryptococcus neoformans* and zygomycetes.

## Aspergillosis

**Causative fungus: *Aspergillus fumigatus*; also *A. flavus*, *A. niger* and occasionally other species.**
Infections caused by *Aspergillus* species are world-wide in distribution and the fungi are ubiquitous in the soil, particularly on decaying vegetable matter. The *Aspergilli* are usually secondary invaders of already diseased or damaged tissues and rarely colonize normal tissues. There are four principal forms of disease:
1) Aspergilloma - a solid ball of fungal mycelium in a pre-existing pulmonary cavity.
2) Allergic bronchopulmonary aspergillosis.
3) Invasive aspergillosis - seen only in immunosuppressed patients.
4) Paranasal aspergillosis - mainly seen in the tropics and caused by *A. flavus*.

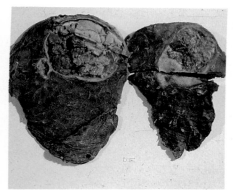

**Fig.131**
Aspergilloma.

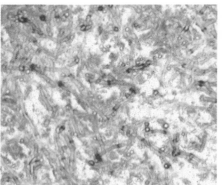

**Fig.132** Section of an aspergilloma showing meshwork of hyphae.
*(Methenamine silver, x256)*

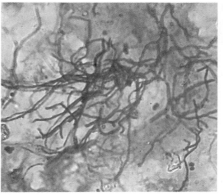

**Fig.133** *Aspergillus* hyphae in sputum. *(Gram, x256)*

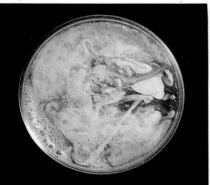

**Fig.134** Bronchial casts or plugs are sometimes found in the sputum from patients with bronchopulmonary aspergillosis.

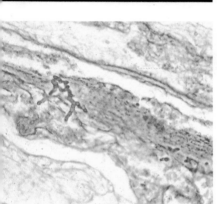

**Fig.135** Section of plug showing Aspergillus filaments. *(Methenamine silver,x256)*

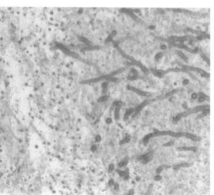

**Fig.136** Section of invasive aspergillosis showing branching hyphae. *(H & E,x256)*

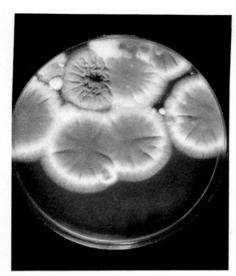

**Fig.137** Culture of *fumigatus* - smoky green colonies develop.

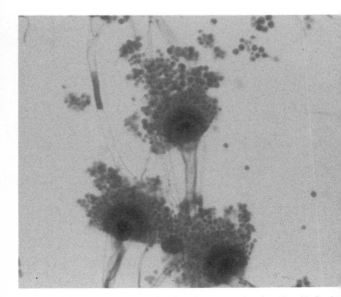

**Fig.138** Microscopical examination shows sporing heads with flask-shaped vesicles; phialides in one series bearing conidia in parallel rows. *(x450)*

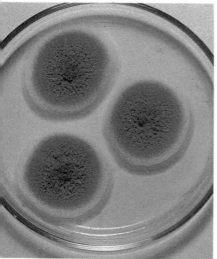

**Fig.139** Culture of *A. flavus* - the colonies are yellow at first, quickly becoming bright to dark yellow/green.

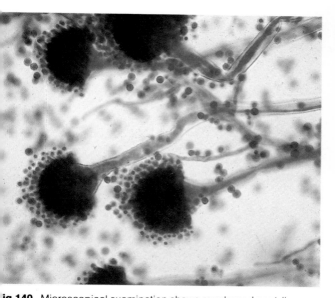

**ig.140** Microscopical examination shows roughened conidiohores with varying sized radiate sporing heads; phialides biseriate earing roughened conidia. *(x384)*

# Blastomycosis

**Causative fungus: *Blastomyces dermatitidis***
The primary lesion occurs in the lungs but cutaneous lesions predominate. The disease was thought to be restricted to the North American continent but cases have now been reported from Africa, Israel and India. The natural habitat of the fungus is not yet known.

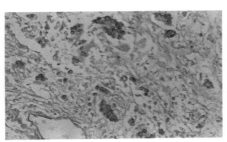

**Fig.141** Section showing thick-walled yeast cells with single broad-based buds. *(PAS,x128)*

*Blastomyces dermatitidis* is a dimorphic fungus:

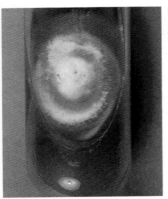

**Fig.142** Culture at 26°C (mycelial form). White to tan cottony colonies are present.

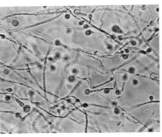

**Fig.143** Microscopical examination shows smooth-walled, round to oval conidia, on the sides of the hyphae. *(x256)*

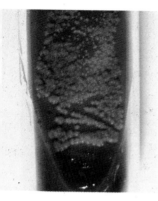

**Fig.144** Culture at 37°C (yeast form). This is a moist, folded creamy colony on brain/heart infusion agar.

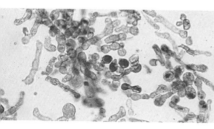

**Fig.145** Thick-walled yeast cells; single buds are attached to the parent cell by a broad base, rapidly developing hyphae. (*PAS, x256*)

## Causative fungus: *Candida albicans*; occasionally other *Candida* species.

Systemic candidosis occurs in debilitated patients and is most commonly seen in patients receiving immunosuppressive therapy. The lesions may be confined to one site or may be widely disseminated. (See also under superficial candidosis.)

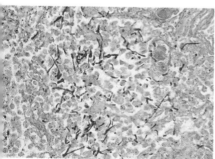

**Fig.146** Section showing hyphae and yeasts of *Candida albicans*. (*PAS,x128*)

# Coccidioidomycosis

## Causative fungus: *Coccidioides immitis*

The infection is usually confined to the lungs and is often subclinical. Chronic pulmonary and disseminated disease may, however, occur. The fungus is endemic in desert-like areas in South Western USA, Mexico and Central and South America where it has been demonstrated in the soil.

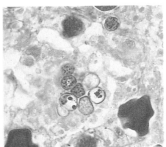

**Fig.147** In tissues, inhaled spores develop into thick-walled spherules. The contents divide to produce small endospores. Mature spherules rupture to release endospores which gradually enlarge and themselves become spherules. (*PAS, x256*)

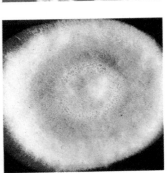

**Fig.148** White cottony, later greyish, mycelial colonies develop at both 26°C and 37°C.

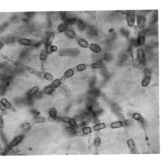

**Fig.149** Microscopical examination shows abundant arthrospores formed by the separation of hyphae, and characteristically alternate with smaller, empty cells. (*x256*)

A safety cabinet should be used for all procedures. Test tubes or screw-capped bottles should be used for cultures

# Cryptococcosis

## Causative fungus: *Cryptococcus neoformans*

The disease is acquired by the inhalation of yeasts and primary infection is in the lungs. Dissemination to the central nervous system frequently occurs and cryptococcal meningitis is the best recognized form of the disease.

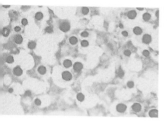

**Fig.150** Section showing encapsulated yeasts. *(Mucicarmine,x128)*

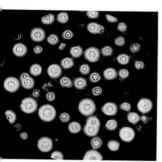

**Fig.151** India ink preparation. This is the best stain to demonstrate the yeast in CSF and other exudates. The yeasts are spherical to oval (5-20 microns in diameter) with single buds and having a wide refractile gelatinous capsule often twice the diameter of the cell.

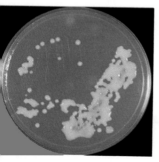

**Fig.152** At both 26°C and 37°C mucoid, shiny cream to tan colonies develop.

Microscopical examination shows yeast cells about 5 microns in diameter, with single buds and capsules. Identification of the culture may be confirmed by biochemical tests.

# Histoplasmosis

### Causative fungus: *Histoplasma capsulatum*

The primary pulmonary infection may be subacute, acute or chronic; occasionally dissemination occurs. The disease is endemic in Mississippi and adjoining states in America, but infections are reported throughout the world. The organism has been demonstrated in soil enriched by chicken and other bird droppings, and bat guano.

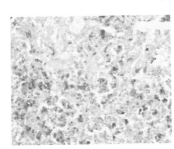

**Fig.153** Section showing small oval yeast cells. (*x256*)

*Histoplasma capsulatum* is a dimorphic fungus;

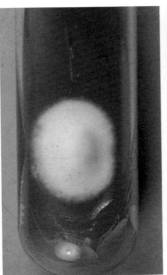

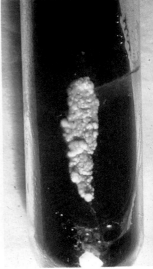

**Fig.154** Culture at 26°C (mycelial form). The colony is white and cottony, later turning a brownish colour.

**Fig.155** Culture at 37°C (yeast form). A moist, folded, creamy colony is seen.

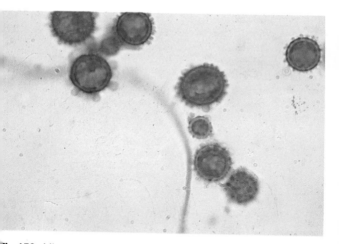

**Fig.156** Microscopical examination shows characteristic thick-walled macroconidia with tuberculate protuberances; small micro-conidia are also present. (*x600*)

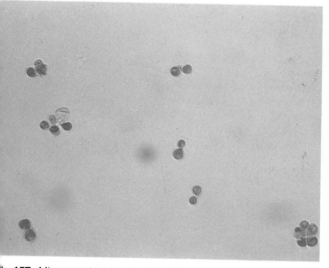

**Fig.157** Microscopical examination shows small yeast cells. (*x600*)

safety cabinet should be used for all procedures. Test tubes or screw-capped bottles should be used for cultures.

# African histoplasmosis

### Causative fungus: *Histoplasma duboisii*

Human cases are confined to Africa and although infection may occur in any tissue of the body, the skin, lymph nodes and bones are most frequently involved.

*Histoplasma duboisii* is a dimorphic fungus and cultures are similar to those of *H. capsulatum*. The yeast form, however, shows large thick-walled yeasts (12 to 15 microns in diameter). Large yeasts are also seen in tissue sections.

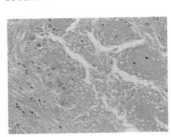

**Fig.158** Section showing large thick-walled yeast cells predominantly in large giant cells. *(PAS,x128)*

Cultures of *H. capsulatum* or *H. duboisii* can only be identified with certainty by infecting laboratory animals and determining the size of tissue forms produced by the isolates.

## Paracoccidioidomycosis

### Causative fungus: *Paracoccidioides brasiliensis*

Primary lesions occur in the lungs and there is a high prevalence of oral lesions. Infections are geographically restricted to South and Central America, but the fungus has not yet been isolated from the natural environment.

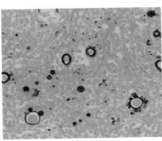

**Fig.159** Section showing yeasts with multiple budding. *(Methanamine silver,x128)*

*Paracoccidioides brasiliensis* is a dimorphic fungus:

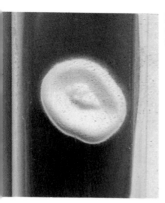

**Fig.160** Culture at 26°C (mycelial form). A white cottony colony develops slowly.

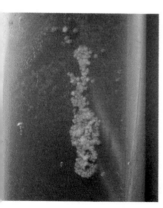

**Fig.161** Culture at 37°C (yeast form). A moist folded creamy colony develops.

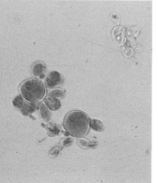

**Fig.162** Microscopical examination shows spherical or oval yeasts with both single and multiple budding. (*x600*)

# Zygomycosis (Phycomycosis, Mucromycosis)

**Causative fungi: *Mucor, Rhizopus, Absidia* and *Saksenaea* species.**

Zygomycosis is an acute and rapidly developing infection in a compromised host. Pulmonary infection is primarily a disease of patients with leukaemia, gastric disease is associated with malnutrition and rhinocerebral infection with diabetes mellitus. The causative organisms are ubiquitous and are found in the soil and on decaying organic debris.

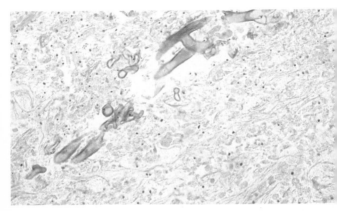

**Fig.163** Section showing broad hyphae sparsely septate and irregularly branched. *(PAS,x96)*

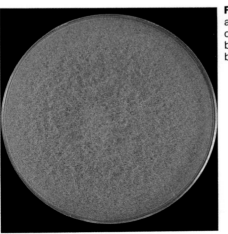

**Fig.164** Colonies are all rapidly growing, cottony, white at first becoming grey to brown.

Microscopical examination:

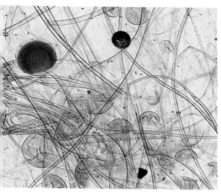

**Fig.165** *Mucor.* Sporangiophores are erect, solitary, branched or simple, arising from the hyphae. Sporangia are globose. No rhizoids or stolons are present.

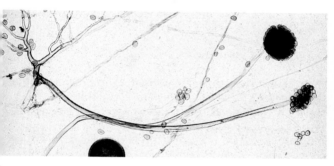

**Fig.166** *Rhizopus.* Sporangiophores are dark, solitary or in clusters and arise opposite rhizoids at a node. Sporangia are globose with flattened bases. *(x256)*

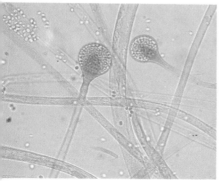

**Fig.167** *Absidia.* Sporangiophores are branched, arising in groups at internodes, with an apical swelling that merges with the pyriform sporangia. Rhizoids when present are not opposite sporangiophores. *(x256)*

# LABORATORY DIAGNOSIS OF MYCOSES

Diagnosis in the laboratory is made by demonstration of the fungus in the skin, exudates or deeper tissues. Isolation of the organism in culture is usually necessary to confirm this and to identify the specific causative fungus. The detection of antibodies and antigens in patients' serum is necessary in the systemic infections, particularly when an early diagnosis is desired, but these tests are generally carried out in specialized laboratories.

The diagnosis of a superficial fungus infection is made by the observation of fungal elements in infected keratin. This can be carried out in a few minutes while the patient is attending the clinic and enough information is usually obtained for treatment to commence. The production of fluorescence under a Wood's lamp (wavelength 3650 Å) will also aid in the detection of certain infected hairs (see Fig.29) and in some other skin conditions, e.g. pityriasis versicolor.

## Collection of material

**Skin** lesions are sampled by scraping with a blunt scalpel and collecting the scales onto clean glass slides. Experience will determine the best material for examination, for instance with a spreading lesion the active periphery is selected (Fig.169). Where vesicles are present, the roof of the blister, cut off with fine pointed scissors, will often reveal abundant hyphae. Vellus hairs from the limbs or face will often show mycelium in the follicle when it may be scanty elsewhere.

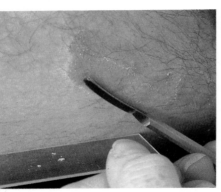

**Fig.169** Collecting skin scrapings.

**Hairs;** A pair of flat-ended forceps is necessary to remove scalp or body hairs but, if they are infected, hair stumps will also be removed easily by scraping with a scalpel. The morphology of the spore arrangement may be more readily preserved if the hairs remain embedded in a scale.

**Nails** are often thickened when infected and clippers are essential to cut off the whole thickness, although subungual debris, removed with a scalpel or probe, may contain fungal elements.

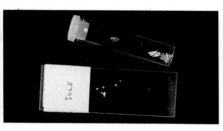

**Fig.170** Skin scales and hairs can be collected between glass slides, but nail clippings will be handled more easily in a small tube or bottle.

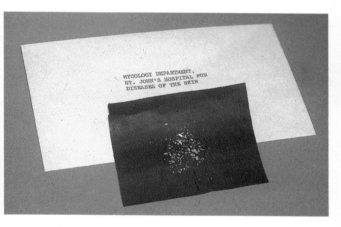

**Fig.171** If any infected material is to be posted to a laboratory, it is recommended that it is placed in folded paper packets. Fungi in keratinous material remain viable for many weeks.

**Mucosae** are sampled with cotton wool swabs. These are placed in transport medium if there is to be any delay before processing.

**Sputum, body fluids, biopsies,** etc. should be collected in sterile containers.

## Observation of fungi in tissues

Samples of skin, hair or nail are placed in a drop of 30% potassium hydroxide (KOH) directly on a microscope slide; after placing a coverslip in position, the specimens can be examined immediately. Softening of the tissue can be hastened by heating gently but hairs should be handled with particular care and allowed to soften without heat so that the arrangement of the spores will not be destroyed.

The incorporation of dimethyl sulphoxide (DMSO) in the potassium hydroxide (DMSO 40ml; distilled water 60ml; KOH 30g) may also help to clarify the specimens.

When examining specimens it is important to ensure that the material has softened adequately and that the intensity of light passing through is not too strong. It is also necessary to alter the focus while scanning the slide.

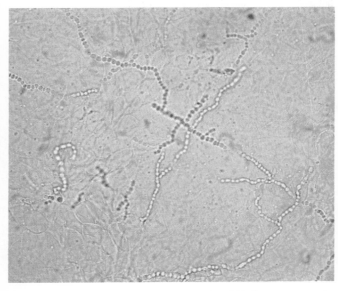

**Fig.172** Dermatophyte hyphae are regular in width, have septa and can show branching. They may be divided into arthrospores. (30% KOH x192)

Unstained preparations are generally satisfactory for the demonstration of fungi in keratin, but chlorazole black E (1) may be added to DMSO to aid in the differentiation of hyphae from common artefacts such as cotton fibres, elastic fibres or 'mosaic fungus'.

73

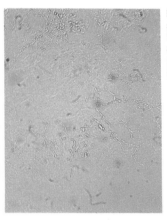

**Fig.173** 'Mosaic fungus' in skin scales. It is an artefact caused by the deposition of cholesterol and other material around the periphery of the epidermal cells. *(30% KOH, x 128)*

If hairs are infected, the size and arrangement of the spores, together with the ability to fluoresce under a Wood's lamp will help towards the identification of the dermatophyte species involved (Figs.175-178).

## Hair Invasion by Dermatophytes

| Species | Spore Arrangement | Size (microns) |
|---|---|---|
| *MICROSPORUM* | | |
| *M. audouinii* | | |
| *M. ferrugineum* | | |
| *M. rivalieri* | Ectothrix* | 2 - 3 |
| *M. canis* | | |
| *M. gypseum* | | |
| *TRICHOPHYTON* | | |
| *T. tonsurans* | | |
| *T. violaceum* | | |
| *T. soudanense* | Endothrix | 4 - 8 |
| *T. gourvilii* | | |
| *T. yaoundei* | | |
| *T. schoenleinii* | Endothrix* | |
| *T. mentagrophytes* | Ectothrix | 3 - 5 |
| *T. verrucosum* | Ectothrix | 5 - 10 |

* = Fluorescence under Wood's lamp

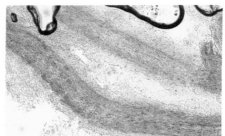

**Fig.174** Small-spored ectothrix invasion of hair by *Microsporum canis.* *(30% KOH, x 64)*

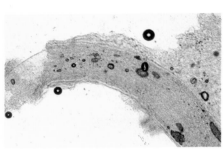

**Fig.175** Large-spored ectothrix invasion of hair by *T. verrucosum.* *(30% KOH, x 64)*

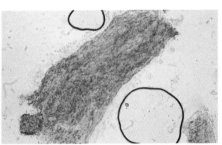

**Fig.176** Endothrix invasion of hair by *T. violaceum.* *(30% KOH x 64)*

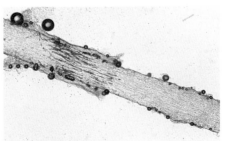

**Fig.177** Favus hair showing hyphae and air spaces infected by *T. schoenleinii.* *(30% KOH, x 64)*

Diagnostic microscopic features shown by fungi other than dermatophytes are illustrated on the relevant pages describing those diseases. Parker's stain, (equal parts of 30% KOH and Parker's blue-black ink) (2) is particularly useful to demonstrate the fungus in scales from pityriasis versicolor as the organism takes up this stain *immediately* (see Fig.66). It may also be helpful to distinguish some non-dermatophyte infections of nails (see Fig.82) but dermatophytes will only take up the blue colour after several hours in the stain.

Smears from **mucosae** may also be examined as unstained wet preparations in saline or KOH but heat fixed preparations may be stained by Gram (see Fig.100) or by periodic acid Schiff (PAS) (Fig.178).

**Pus, exudates and body fluids** may be spun down and the deposit examined for the presence of yeasts, filaments or spherules either unstained or after staining by Gram, PAS, methenamine silver, Giemsa or mucicarmine according to the disease suspected. For cryptococcosis, and particularly when any CSF material is being examined, an India ink preparation should be included (see Fig.151).

Sections from **biopsy specimens** should be stained using the above stains as appropriate.

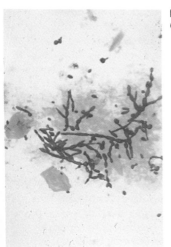

**Fig.178** Smear showing *Candida* stained by PAS. (x256)

# Culture of specimens

Petri dishes are very satisfactory for the culture of fungi but cotton wool plugged tubes may also be used. Screw capped bottles are essential when hazardous species such as *Histoplasma capsulatum* and *Coccidioides immitis* are suspected but they do not allow for the maximum development of spores and pigments which are necessary for the identification of many species.

**Sabouraud Dextrose Agar** (SDA) is the medium most commonly used (Peptone-preferably mycological, 1%, Dextrose 4%, Agar 1.5%,pH 5.6). A broad spectrum antibacterial antibiotic, e.g. chloramphenicol (0.005%) is incorporated and the medium can be made selective for dermatophytes by adding cycloheximide (0.05%) (3) to inhibit contaminating fungi. However, when attempting to isolate yeasts or any other non-dermatophytes, cyclo- heximide should be excluded or a duplicate series of plates used. Both chloramphenicol and cycloheximide may be added to the medium before sterilizing.

Sabouraud Dextrose Agar is available commercially in dehydrated form from several sources, but as the morph- ology of the fungi, particularly the production of pig- ments, will vary according to the source of the medium, it is advisable to confine supplies to one company. This also applies to the nature of the peptone if the medium is prepared from individual ingredients. Other dehydrated media are available which include the antibiotics mentioned above either incorporated in the powder, Mycobiotic Agar (Difco, Gibco) and Mycosel (BBL) or with the antibiotics in separate vials, Dermasel (Oxoid).

A medium which will aid a non-specialist laboratory to differentiate dermatophytes from other fungi is Derma- tophyte Test Medium (DTM) (4). A change in pH produced by the proteolytic activity of dermatophytes is demonstrated by the incorporation of phenol red in the medium. A change from yellow to red indicates the presence of a dermatophyte. The medium can be used for primary cultures if antibiotics are included and has a particular use in identifying dermatophyte isolations in large field studies (Fig.179). It is available commercially.

A richer medium such as Brain Heart Infusion Agar may be necessary to isolate fungi causing deep mycoses, parti- cularly for the yeast phases of the dimorphic species.

The medium should be poured to give thick plates

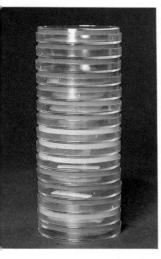

**Fig.179** Skin specimens on DTM; the red colour indicates the growth of dermtophytes.

(25ml per plate) and allowed to dry by leaving at room temperature overnight, so minimising drying out of the agar throughout the long incubation time.

Hairs, small fragments of skin, or nails clipped into as small pieces as possible are placed on the surface of the agar with the aid of a straight needle and pressed in to the surface to make a good contact.

Biopsy material should be ground or cut up into small pieces to give numerous inocula, and for the culture of blood, vented blood culture bottles with biphasic media are recommended.

Incubation at room temperature is adequate for the isolation of dermatophytes but 26°C to 28°C is preferred. Cultures may be identified after 10 to 14 days' incubation. Yeasts and Aspergilli may be isolated at 37°C on plates incubated for 2 to 10 days. When a dimorphic fungus is suspected, cultures should be placed at both 26°C and 37°C in order to isolate the filamentous and yeast phases of the organisms respectively. Plates or bottles of culture from deeper tissues should be incubated for up to 3 to 4 weeks according to the disease suspected.

Scalps may be sampled for culture using a brush technique which is a useful method to survey siblings and contacts of infected children and also suspected pets in the household.

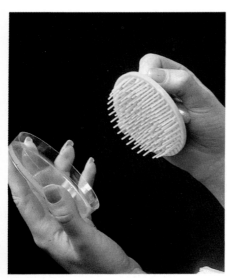

**Fig.180** A commercially available massage brush is pressed into a petri dish containing medium after a vigorous brushing of the scalp.

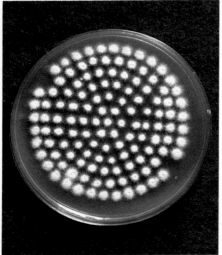

**Fig.181** Clinically infected children produce fungal colonies from many points of the brush.

# Identification of isolates

Fungi are usually identified by the recognition of morphological features and, to a lesser degree, by their biochemical properties. Macroscopic features such as the texture of the colony, the surface colour and production of pigments seen on the reverse side of the plate may be diagnostic.

To examine under the microscope, a small portion of the culture is teased out in a drop of lactophenol cotton blue (Phenol crystals 20g, Lactic acid 20ml, Glycerol 40ml, Distilled water 20ml; phenol crystals are dissolved by gently heating and Cotton blue 0.075g added). If sporulation is adequate, a strip of sellotape pressed on to the culture surface and subsequently placed on a drop of stain and pressed onto the slide will reveal the spore arrangement satisfactorily (Fig.182).

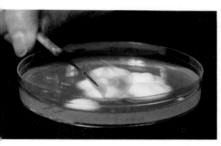

**Fig.182** Examination of culture using sellotape.

A slide culture prepared by inoculating each side of a block of agar on a slide is more time consuming but may be necessary to encourage sporulation (Fig.183). After sufficient growth has developed, the agar block is discarded and stained preparations made of the growth remaining on the slide and coverslip.

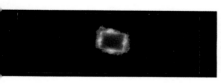

**Fig.183** Slide culture.

In some cultures (e.g. *T.schoenleinii)*, the diagnostic features can be seen by placing the culture plate directly on the stage of the microscope and examining the reverse side directly with a low power objective.

## Additional tests used in identification of dermatophytes.

### 1. Urease Test

Urea Agar Base (Difco) is prepared in solid form and dispensed in tubes. The ability of fungi to attack urea and change the colour of the medium from straw to red within 7 days will distinguish floccose forms of *T. rubrum* from *T. mentagrophytes* (Fig.184) and *T. megninii*, and also *T. erinacei* from *T. mentagrophytes*. A positive reaction is shown by *T. mentagrophytes* and *T. megninii* while *T. rubrum* and *T. erinacei* are both urease negative.

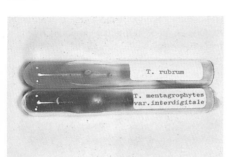

**Fig.184** *T. rubrum* - urease negative; *T. mentagrophytes* -urease positive.

### 2. Penetration of hair in vitro

The ability to produce transverse perforations in sterile human hair will distinguish *T. mentagrophytes* from *T. rubrum*. Short lengths of human hair are sterilized and added to distilled water in a petri dish with 2 to 3 drops of 10% yeast extract. After inoculation the hairs are incubated for up to 4 weeks and examined at intervals for the formation of wedge shaped perforations which are formed by *T. mentagrophytes* (Fig.185). No perforations are formed by *T. rubrum*.

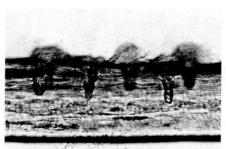

**Fig.185** Hair penetration by *T. mentagrophytes.* (x256)

## 3. Growth on rice grains

A few grains of rice are placed in a small flask or bottle, covered with distilled water and sterilized. The test organism is inoculated onto the surface of the rice and incubated for 10 to 14 days. This test differentiates *M. audouinii*, which will not grow on the rice grains, from *M. canis* or *M. gypseum*, both of which produce thick growth (Fig.186). This medium also encourages the production of characteristic macroconidia in atypical isolates of *M. canis*.

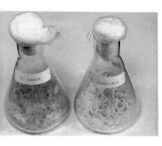

**Fig.186** Growth on rice grains by *M. canis*; no growth by *M. audounii*.

## 4. Pigment production on 1% peptone agar

*Microsporum persicolor* will develop a pink colour on the surface when grown on agar containing 1% peptone after 7 to 14 days. *Trichophyton mentagrophytes* will not produce any surface pigment (Fig.187).

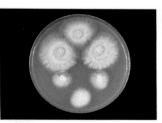

**Fig.187** *M. persicolor* (top) and *T. mentagrophytes* (bottom) on 1% peptone agar.

## 5. Nutritional requirements

The series of Trichophyton Agars No.1 - 7 (Difco) can be used to differentiate some *Trichophyton* species by demonstrating the requirement of growth factors. Examples are *T. equinum* which requires nicotinic acid, *T. violaceum* requires thiamine and *T. megninii* requires histidine.

## Physiological tests for yeast identification

The principal tests for the identification of yeasts involve the investigation of isolates for their ability to ferment sugars and also to assimilate various sources of carbohydrates and nitrates. However, commercial identification kits which give sufficient information to identify most isolates encountered in a medical laboratory are available.

The Urease test as previously described is also useful in yeast identification. *Cryptococcus* species can be confirmed by a positive urease reaction, whereas most *Candida* and *Saccharomyces* species are urease negative.

## FURTHER READING

Chandler, F.W., Kaplan, W. and Ajello, L. (1980) A Colour Atlas and Textbook of the Histopathology of Mycotic Diseases. Wolfe Medical Publications Ltd.
Howard, D.H. (editor) (1983) Fungi Pathogenic for Humans and Animals: Part B Pathogenicity and Detection; 1. Marcel Dekker, Inc.
McGinnis, M.R. (1980) Laboratory Handbook of Medical Mycology. Academic Press.
Rippon, J.W. (1982) Medical Mycology - The Pathogenic Fungi and the Pathogenic Actinomycetes. 2nd edition. W.B. Saunders Company.

## REFERENCES

(1) Burke, W.A. and Jones, B.E. (1984) A simple stain for rapid office diagnosis of fungus infections of the skin. Arch. Derm., **120**, 1519.
(2) Cohen, M.N. (1958) An easy office procedure for staining superficial fungi with fountain pen ink. Bull. Sch. Med. Univ. Md., **43**, 20.
(3) Georg, L.K. (1953) Use of cycloheximide medium for isolation of dermatophytes from clinical materials. Arch. Derm., **67**, 355.
(4) Taplin, D., Zaias, N., Rebell, G. and Blank, H. (1969) Isolation and recognition of dermatophytes on a new medium (DTM). Arch. Derm., **99**, 203.

# Index

Entries in **bold** refer to Fig. numbers